The Vitamii

How to Cure Common Health Problems and Have Optimal Health

Introduction

Nutrition forms the basis of our being. Experts believe that no matter how much physical activity you engage in or how hard you work out, you can never bring your body to its optimal functioning condition if you do not provide the body with the nutrition that it requires. 75% of our physical being is made from the kind of food that we eat. The rest of it is determined by the amount we exercise, the amount of sleep that we get and the amount of relaxation that the body gets. With these four factors in balance it is possible for every individual to lead the healthiest life.

When we discuss nutrition, we normally talk about food groups like proteins, carbohydrates and fats. However, unknown to most of us, there are several nutrients that actually give meaning to the consumption of the major food groups. Without these other nutrients, it is impossible for the body to carry out processes that break down and utilize these food groups. These additional nutrients that make our body function better include vitamins and minerals. They are perhaps the most neglected food groups although they are essential in helping our body function properly.

Coming to the vitamins, we have all heard of the glorious benefits of vitamin B and vitamin C. While one of them is great at regulating the heat in the body, the other is very important in providing immunity against common health problems. There are four more vitamins that are mandatory to maintain our body functions and also facilitate these functions. These vitamins are Vitamin A, Vitamin D, Vitamin E and Vitamin K. They are responsible for specific functions but work in unison to ensure that the body functions at its best.

In this book, I would like to focus upon the most beneficial but the most overlooked Vitamin- Vitamin D. Also known as the sunshine vitamin, this is one of the most important vitamins responsible for_ maintaining the very framework of our body-the skeletal system. Without this vitamin, no matter how much calcium you consume, you will not be able to improve bone health or even achieve the amount of calcium that your body requires to function properly. Although Vitamin D is a very tiny organic compound, it regulates functions in almost all parts of the body. This is what gives vitamin D a very unique quality.

The best part about vitamin D is that it is the easiest vitamin to obtain and synthesize in the body. Still, vitamin D deficiency is an epidemic that has swept the entire globe. The only reason for this is the ignorance in people and in health professionals as well about the uses and the benefits of Vitamin D.

This book explores all the nuances about Vitamin D. From the different forms of vitamin D to the several sources of Vitamin D, this book covers just almost everything that you need to know about Vitamin D. The next time you need any vital information about this vital nutrient, all you have to do is flip through the pages.

I hope you enjoy reading this book. Thank you for downloading it.

Chapter 1: Vitamin D: The Discovery

We have all heard about the several benefits of vitamins in our diet. Vitamin D, especially, is extremely important for our body to be able to utilize the calcium that we take in. The most interesting thing about nutrients is their history. How did we discover what our body needs? Who was responsible for pointing out the functions of these nutrients in our bodies? Considering that they are tiny molecules ~~that they are such tiny molecules~~, the knowledge that we have acquired about them is quite astonishing. The discovery of vitamin D is no different. This story is particularly interesting as Vitamin D is not even an essential dietary vitamin.

 Let us take a tour through the history of Vitamin D and learn about the people responsible for the elaborate knowledge that we have today.

Discovery through cure for Rickets

Until the early 19th century, Rickets was a common disease among children. Cod liver oil was prescribed as the only cure for this disease as vitamin D was still unknown. Although there were several details available about the causes and the cures for Rickets, none of them were accurate. In the 17th century, a detailed description of rickets was created by

Francis Glisson in the "Treatise of the Rickets". Sadly, there was no understanding of the actual cause. All they knew back then was that rickets could not be genetically inherited and was not contagious. He did point out possible nutritional causes and came as close as over feeding and indigestion.

The biggest breakthrough in the understanding of the role of vitamins in nutrition came from the work of Frederick Hopkins. He conducted several studies on the oxidation and reduction processes that occur within the cells to produce energy. It was through his studies with animal feeding that Hopkins discovered the role of nutrients in our health. He conducted a series of experiments where animals were fed pure proteins, fats, carbohydrates, minerals and water. He recorded that just these nutrients did not support their growth. So, logically, there had to be other nutrients that made growth possible. He named them "Accessory Food Factors". This is what we know today as Vitamins.

Once they learnt about the existence of these essential food factors, scientists began to conduct detailed studies in an attempt to isolate and understand these factors thoroughly.

Scientist McCollum and his team were among the first ones to approach the study of essential dietary factors scientifically. It was in the year 1914 that they isolated "fat soluble factor A" from butter. This factor was also able to prevent xerophthalmia in rats. This factor was nothing but the Vitamin A that we know of today.

Now, there was a new piece of information available. These factors were fat soluble. With this came the biggest breakthrough in the discovery of Vitamin D. In the year 1919, Edwards Mellanby conducted a study with puppies. He gave the puppies a very low fat diet with some milk. This induced a bone disease that was very similar to rickets. Through his studies, X ray examinations, histology and even bone calcium assay he discovered that the bone constitution in these puppies was similar to that of children with rickets. He provided these puppies with yeast and orange juice which provided vitamin B and C respectively. Even after continuing with this diet for over 4 months. However, when these puppies were given butterfat, the condition diminished. This led to the conclusion that either fat soluble factor A or something very similar to it was responsible for the prevention of rickets.

To gain more clarity, McCollum conducted other studies with cod liver oil. Oxidation of cod liver oil was able to cure rickets in rats but was not able to prevent xerophthalmia. The only obvious result of this was the discovery of another factor that existed in cod liver oil along with fat soluble factor A. While fat soluble factor A was destroyed with oxidation, this other factor remained intact.

By then, fat soluble factor A was known as vitamin A, the water soluble factors were known as vitamin B and the anti-scurvy factor was known as vitamin C. So, this new factor was called Vitamin D!

Another Cure for Rickets- Sunlight

While studies were being conducted to reveal this additional factor, there was one tremendous discovery about a cure for rickets- UV rays. Although it was a popular belief that staying out in the sun and getting some fresh air helped cure rickets, there was no scientific basis for this until scientist Huldschinsky carried out experiments in the year 1919. In his experiment, he allowed children with rickets to be exposed to a quartz mercury lamp that emitted UV rays for 20 minutes for a stretch of 2 months. The X-rays of these children revealed better calcium deposits. During this period, these children were not given any supplements and were not even exposed to direct sunlight.

Now, things got more interesting in the path towards the discovery of Vitamin D. There was a component in cod liver oil and butterfat that was entirely different from Vitamin A. At the same time, rickets was also cured with the help of UV rays stimulation. There were several tests conducted to understand this phenomenon.

But, people still did not have a complete understanding of this additional factor. Sure, it was called Vitamin D, but what did it look like? What exactly was it? One important discovery came from the study of cholesterol extracted from the brain of rats. This substance when activated became anti-rachitic. So cholesterol was assumed to be the precursor of this substance. Further investigations revealed that an impurity found in cholesterol could be the pro-vitamin that scientists were in search of. So it was not cholesterol but that impurity which was the precursor of Vitamin D. This impurity also had chemical properties similar to steroids.

It was the work of scientists Windaus and Hess that revealed the pro-vitamin. They prepared 30 different steroids from plant sources to check which one of them became anti-rachitic upon irradiation. They found the answer in ergosterol which was a type of steroid found in the ergot fungi. The structure of this steroid was clearly presented by Windaus and Thiele. For this work of his, Windaus even went on to win the Nobel Prize.

Now, the question that remained was; ergosterol did not occur in animals, so how do we get Vitamin D? This problem was solved in the year 1937 when Windaus isolated a certain compound from hog's skin. This compound was also found in animal skin and human skin and certain foods like whole milk. This compound was created from cholesterol and when it was irradiated, it produced vitamin D-3. With further thermal and photochemical reactions, Vitamin D was produced in the skin.

We will get into the details of the formation of Vitamin D in our body and its benefits to our health. For now, I simply want you to be able to appreciate the effort that has been put into discovering and understanding the several nutrients that we take for granted. Vitamins, especially, are neglected the most owing to a lack of information about their role in our growth and development.

Vitamin D and its several forms are more important to us than we think. This E-book takes you through all the details that you will need to lead a healthier life.

Chapter 2: Vitamin D: The Most Overlooked Vitamin

When we think Vitamin D, we think sunlight. Now, just to clarify any doubts, Vitamin D is not found in sunlight. In the presence of Sunlight and UV rays, Vitamin D is synthesized in our skin. Similarly, there are several misconceptions about Vitamin D that make it a highly overlooked vitamin.

To begin with, the name given to Vitamin D, "The Bone Vitamin" was itself quite limiting in understanding the importance of this Vitamin. It was only due to extensive research by significant people like Dr. Michael Holick that the real importance of Vitamin D has become known to health professionals across the globe.

According to the data obtained from this research, every single cell in our body contains Vitamin D receptors. This is an alarming revelation as the dose that is normally available to us, is much lesser than what our body actually requires. And not obtaining the optimal levels of vitamin D means that we are putting ourselves at risk to several diseases besides the common ones arising from vitamin D deficiency.

From weak bones to diseases like Alzheimer's, vitamin D has an important role to play. Let me give you an example to make this easier to understand. We normally associate an alteration in blood sugar levels to diabetes. And, as expected, our diet is focused at controlling sugar intake to reduce the risk of diabetes. However, research states that even a person with normal sugar levels is susceptible to type II diabetes if the intake of vitamin D is not optimum. In fact, you are 91% more likely to progress to active diabetes type II if you do not have enough vitamin D intake. This is because your system develops a resistance to insulin, doubling the risk of a progression.

If you do not get enough Vitamin D, you are 20 times more at risk of developing Alzheimer's and dementia!

These are just a few examples. There are several other conditions that you can develop if your tissues are not given the amount of Vitamin D that they require. Still, deficiency of this vitamin is an epidemic that has swept the globe.

Not many physicians check the level of vitamin D in our body as a standard practice. This itself is a big let down in the field of healthcare. This vitamin acts as your first level of defense against several diseases that are constantly lurking around. It is not just one or two organs that are at risk, the list of possible diseases due to vitamin D deficiency spans every system in our body.

The good news, however, is that restoring the optimal level of vitamin D in our body is not very difficult. It is not only easy, it is also inexpensive. As you will learn from the following chapters, vitamin D is actually a vitamin of great convenience!

Chapter 3: Vitamin D Deficiency: A Global Epidemic

Although the apparent benefits of Vitamin D are so many, its deficiency is a raging global epidemic. Close to 1 billion people, globally, do not get the amount of Vitamin D that their body requires to perform at its best.

If you trace your own routine, how much time do you really get outdoors? We are usually cooped up in offices for a good 6-8 hours each day. So, with the lack of adequate sunlight, are we at least compensating with our diet? Well, how many of us know of good vitamin D sources besides sunlight? It is no wonder that we are all susceptible to so many health hazards that vary in their intensity and effect.

In America alone, over 64% of the population does not receive enough vitamin D for the tissues to perform at their best. Out of this number, 39% of them actually suffer from deficiencies while the remaining 24% does not get the required amount of vitamin D.

The question is how do we measure deficiency? For our bodies to function normally, we need to keep the vitamin D level in our blood at least 30ng/ml. To function optimally, we need to bring these numbers up to 50 ng/ml.

When a person is said to have an insufficient intake of vitamin D, the level is about *between* 21 or 29 ng/ml. However, any number below 20 ng/ml is considered a deficiency.

There are several sources of vitamin D that we will discuss about in detail in the following chapter. You can also read about the tests that you can undergo to have the vitamin D level in your body determined. At least then you will know how far behind your body is from optimum nutrition or, hopefully, how close it is.

Chapter 4: What exactly is Vitamin D?

Before we move on to other details of Vitamin D like why it is important for our body and how we can obtain it, let us understand what it actually is. What does it look like and in what forms does it exist?

Like we saw in the discovery process of vitamin D, it is a form of steroid that is known as a secosteroid. Now, steroids are made of several carbon rings. When these are broken, the compound obtained is known as a secosteroid.

Vitamin D is popularly known as the 'sunshine vitamin' as it can be synthesized in our skin when we receive enough sunlight. The cholesterol in the skin is utilized to produce active compounds of vitamin D that our body can use. The primary role of vitamin D in our body is to increase the absorption of iron, magnesium, phosphate, calcium and zinc.

Not really a vitamin?

One interesting thing about Vitamin D is that although it is called a vitamin, it is quite different from the other vitamins that we consume. It does not really qualify as an essential dietary vitamin. Now, this does not mean that vitamin D is not essential for our diet; it only means that vitamin D is not produced in adequate amounts within our body. While we are able to make small amounts of vitamins within our body, it is not adequate to fulfill the requirement of our tissues.

Of course, like any other vitamin, Vitamin D was discovered in order to understand the nutritional deficit in children suffering from rickets. Also, like any other vitamin, Vitamin D is also found in supplements and is also added to staple foods like milk.

Types of Vitamin D

The name Vitamin D is given to a compound that exists in several forms. This name is like a collective term for five other compounds that exist under it. The five types of Vitamin D are:

- Vitamin D1 (scientifically made from ergocalciferol and lumisterol)
- Vitamin D2- (scientifically known as ergosterol)
- Vitamin D3- (scientifically known as cholecalciferol)
- Vitamin D4- (22- dihydroergoclciferol)
- Vitamin D5- (sitocalciferol)

Although the scientific names seem too fancy, the difference between the five forms of vitamin D lies in their structure.

Although the basic structure is the same, a few chemical bonds make a big difference.

The only two types of vitamin that are relevant to us are Vitamin D2 and Vitamin D3. These compounds are usually found in all the vitamin D supplements that we consume. They are the active forms of vitamin D that our body is capable of metabolizing. Together, they are known as calciferol. However, they can also be manufactured separately.

The next time you buy a vitamin D supplement, take a moment to look at the contents. Usually, Vitamin D2 or vitamin D3 is listed as the primary ingredient.

The difference between Vitamin D2 and D3 is in the side chain. Like I mentioned before, all these forms of vitamin D contain a basic structure. Chemical groups that are attached to this basic structure are known as side chains. In Vitamin D2, there is a double bond between the 22nd and the 23rd carbon atom with a hydroxide molecule attached to the 24th carbon atom. In vitamin D3, there is no double bond and hydroxide molecule. This simple difference in the structure makes them entirely different from each other. The way they are synthesized in the body and their reaction to various body processes makes them significantly different.

Unlike Vitamin D3, vitamin D2 is not produced in animals. This is because vitamin D2 is derived from a fungus called ergot fungus which is usually produced by yeasts, fungi and other invertebrates. For the production of vitamin D2, the irradiation of a particular compound known as ergosterol is necessary. In vertebrates, this important precursor is missing which makes it impossible for them to synthesize it. However, vitamin D2 is produced synthetically and added to several vitamin substitutes that we consume.

Vitamin D3 on the other hand can be produced in our skin. A derivative of cholesterol, known as 7-dehydraocholesterol, is the precursor for the formation of this vitamin. When ultraviolet rays act upon this compound, Vitamin D3 is produced. 90% of our vitamin D requirement is fulfilled by vitamin D3. It is also found in several animal products like milk. It can also be obtained from cod liver oil and some types of fish.

There is a lot of debate about the efficiency of vitamin D2 in our body. Although it is recommended as a dietary supplement, health professionals do not completely agree that this form can replace vitamin D3 entirely. The only common factor between the two forms is that they become active only with irradiation from ultraviolet rays of the sun.

Let us now compare these two forms of vitamins to understand which one is a better supplement.

Vitamin D3 or D2?

If you are purchasing a Vitamin D supplement over the counter, you will find either vitamin D3 supplements or vitamin D2 supplements. Just to remind you again, Vitamin D3 is called cholecalciferol and vitamin D2 is called ergocalciferol. So, when you look for the primary ingredient in the contents chart, you will either have the generic name or the scientific name listed in it. Now, although vitamin D2 is highly accepted as a great supplement, several experts believe that vitamin D3 is a far better option. There are several logical reasons that have led scientists to believe that vitamin D3 has a lot more benefits because of the way our body reacts to it. In my personal research, too, I have found that vitamin D3 is easier for our body to utilize and is a more natural form of vitamin that is available to us.

Here are some valid reasons that make me choose to believe that D3 is the better way to go:

- **Easiest available form of Vitamin D:** The human body is able to synthesize a small amount of vitamin D when sunlight falls on the skin. This is because a certain derivative of cholesterol that is present in our skin gets converted into cholecalciferol or Vitamin D3. So, when we make vitamin D in our body it is in the form of Vitamin D3. As a result, it is obvious that this is the most natural form available. Hence, it is easy for our body to consume.

- **Lesser traces in Blood:** When we consume vitamin D2, there are chances that it will remain in our blood stream for a longer time. As I mentioned before, every single cell in our body has a vitamin receptor. It is easier for vitamin D3 to bind itself to these receptors in comparison to vitamin D2. The advantage with this is that the toxicity of Vitamin D3 is far lesser than vitamin D2. We know that overconsumption of vitamins can create havoc in our system. So, Vitamin D3 is a safer option, if you consume a higher dosage unknowingly.

- **More Potent Form:** In comparison to vitamin D2, Vitamin D3 is more potent. This means that when a person is suffering from deficiency, consuming vitamin D3 will produce better results. There may also be instances when the vitamin D levels in the body need to be lowered. For instance, in obese people, vitamin D concentration in the blood might have to be reduced. In such cases, too, Vitamin D3 is a better option as it is more potent and also easier to metabolize.

- **Better Shelf Life:** Storing Vitamin D3 is easier in comparison to Vitamin D2 as the shelf life is higher. The Vitamin D3 found in supplements will remain active for longer periods of time. Several tests have been conducted to test the effect of humidity and temperature on these supplements. The results have been in the favor of Vitamin D3 in most cases. As a result, several fortified foods contain a lower amount of vitamin D2 than what is advertised on the pack. There are chances that this is true for the supplements as well. This means that you might be consuming a much lower amount than what you think you are consuming. So, if you are taking supplements to replenish the amount of vitamin D in your body, vitamin D2 supplements will be less helpful.

In addition to these four obvious reasons, health experts recommend Vitamin D3 supplements because there is more clinical evidence available to support the effect of Vitamin D3. There are very few clinical trials available to support the role of Vitamin D2 in improving our bone structure and strength. Also, Vitamin D2 is derived from fungus/yeast when certain foods are subjected to ultraviolet rays. This is not the most natural form that our body will be able to respond to. Hence, it is always better that you opt for Vitamin D3 supplements. However, vegans and vegetarians who do not consume animal products may find vitamin D2 more appealing.

Chapter 5: Production and Metabolism of Vitamin D in our Body

Vitamin D production in our skin

Any chemical reaction that takes place in the presence of sunlight is called a photochemical reaction. So, the synthesis of vitamin D in our skin is also a photochemical reaction. These chemical reactions are quite complex but I will make it as simple as I can to help you understand how beautifully our body maintains a balanced vitamin D concentration.

Now, for any element to be produced there needs to be a precursor. Think of the precursor as the tomatoes in your ketchup. Without these tomatoes, how will you make the ketchup? Similarly, the precursor for Vitamin D in our body is 7- dehydrocholesterol. This is a derivative of the cholesterol that is already present in our body. This is available in large quantities in our body. With about 30 minutes of exposure of the entire body to sunlight, about 10,000 to 20,000 IU (International Units) of Vitamin D is produced. When 7-dehydrocholesterol reacts with a certain wavelength of UV rays available from sunlight, it is broken down into cholecalciferol, which is Vitamin D3.

Now, you might wonder what might happen if we are in the sun for too long. Is there a chance of Vitamin D toxicity? Well, not with the amazing design of the Human Body. Our body has been programmed to degenerate the vitamin D3 produced in the skin just as fast as it is created. This maintains the equilibrium necessary.

Our skin consists of two layers- the dermis, which is the inner layer and the epidermis, which is the outer layer. Usually the epidermis is a very thin layer except in parts of the body like our sole and palms. In the thicker sections, the epidermis contains five layers. Vitamin D is usually produced in the epidermis. In areas where it is divided into five layers, it is the innermost layer where vitamin D is produced.

Just like humans, most vertebrates are able to produce vitamin D in their skin. I would like to mention one more marvel of nature while we are discussing the production of vitamin D in animals. Unlike humans, whose skin is directly exposed to the UV rays necessary to synthesize vitamin D, most vertebrates have a layer of fur or feather. In these animals, the oil secreted by the skin generates vitamin D. And, when the animals groom themselves, they orally consume vitamin D.

I have always been amazed at how one of the easiest vitamins to obtain is deficient in most people. There are several reasons that lead to the global epidemic of vitamin D deficiency. Before we delve into that, let us look at how the vitamin D3 produced in the skin reaches the rest of the body. The understanding of the metabolism of Vitamin D3 will help you understand how calcium is related to Vitamin D3.

Chapter 6: Metabolism of Vitamin D

The first step towards the utilization of any nutrient in the body is its activation. The nutrient is converted, through a series of chemical reactions, into a substance that our body can recognize and utilize. The biologically active form of vitamin is called calcitriol. Once the Vitamin D3 that is synthesized in our skin is transferred to our bloodstream. From there, it is carried over to the liver.

In the liver, a hydroxide molecule (OH) gets added to the cholecalciferol (Vitamin D3), converting it into an element which is known as calcidol. The calcidol that is circulated in the blood is then carried over to the kidneys where it is converted into calcitriol, the biologically active form. This binds itself to the vitamin D receptors found in cells. This is how it gets carried to various organs that require vitamin D.

This biologically active form of vitamin D is also synthesized by our immune system. The calcitriol produced in our immune system, however, plays an entirely different role. It is only used locally by the immune system to stimulate reactions against microorganisms that invade our body. So, you see, vitamin D has several functions besides being the bone vitamin.

Even the vitamins that are ingested directly go through the same process. All these reactions are speeded up by several enzymes that our body secretes. In the first series of reactions that take place in our liver, an enzyme called vitamin D 25-hydroxylase is produced by the cells in the liver. Once the calcitriol is carried to the kidneys, it is acted upon by enzymes known as 25-hydroxyvitamin D3 and 1-alpha hydroxylase. These enzymes are produced almost instantaneously when the presence of Vitamin D3 in the body is detected.

The interesting thing here is that all the chemical reactions responsible for the proper utilization of the vitamin D3 in our body are controlled by two tiny glands present on the either side of our thyroid glands. They are known as the parathyroid glands. They produce a hormone called the parathyroid hormone which regulates the amount of enzymes required for the chemical reactions to take place. Another important trigger for the production of this hormone is the reduction in the level of calcium or phosphate in the body. This is for faster synthesis of Vitamin D3 which allows the levels to be restored.

One important thing that I would like to point out here is that all the bodily functions responsible for the utilization of vitamin D are triggered by the presence of vitamin D3. Therefore, it is important for me to stress on the importance of Vitamin D3 supplements in comparison to any other variety available in the market, if you are planning to take vitamin D supplements.

How does vitamin D work in our body?

After the vitamin D3 that is either synthesized in the body or orally consumed has been converted into a biologically active form, it has several things to do. Like any other nutrient, it is consumed with a very specific purpose. So once it is converted, what exactly happens to this nutrient?

There are several target organs in our body that the vitamin D3 needs to be redirected to. Every organ is made of several cells that contain a central mass called the nucleus or the nuclei. This is the same little space where the entire DNA is present. In this nucleus, a certain binding protein called the Vitamin D Receptor is located.

Now, what exactly does this Vitamin D receptor do? Let me give you a simple example to make that easier to understand. Let us suppose you have to go to a mall about 10 blocks away from your house, you would probably take your car or the bus to get there. Assuming that you are the active vitamin D molecule, the car or the bus is the Vitamin D Receptor. It is the vehicle or the transport that takes the vitamin D to various organs in our body. Surprisingly, these Vitamin D Receptors are expressed not only in the cells of our skeletal system but also in the cells of the brain, the breasts, the gonads, the skin, the heart and the prostate. It is through the activation of these vitamin D Receptors that the levels of calcium and phosphorous are maintained in the blood. Of course, there are hormones like the parathyroid hormones and also calcitonin that assist this process.

So, how exactly is Vitamin D responsible for the maintenance of calcium and phosphorous balance in our body? All the constructive business in our body is taken care of by proteins. They are not called the building blocks of our body for no reason. As soon as the biologically active form of Vitamin D binds itself to the Vitamin D Receptors, certain transport proteins in the intestines also become active. These transport proteins are responsible for the absorption of calcium in our intestines. The calcium that has been absorbed by our intestines are reabsorbed by the cells in our bones.

Thus, bone formation is promoted by the intake of an adequate amount of vitamin D. There is a very delicate balance that is maintained in our body. While some hormones are meant to alert the body about a lack of certain nutrients, it is also equally important for us to fulfill the request raised by these hormones for them to continue to perform properly. Similarly, for the parathyroid hormone to function properly, we must ensure that calcium and phosphorus are available to the body.

So, you see, even if you are recommended regular calcium supplements, they are entirely useless if you do not have the right amount of Vitamin D in your body. Of course, there are several organs that require vitamin D. quite obviously; these organs perform some critical functions when vitamin D is available in the required quantity. In the following chapter, we will discuss in detail, the role vitamin D in our body.

Chapter 7: The Role of Vitamin D in our Body

Continuous research in the field of medicine and nutrition has helped health experts understand that Vitamin D is not restricted in its function towards our skeletal system. There are several target organs in our body that require a regular dose of vitamin D. It is interesting to know that this nutrient that we give such little credit to is actually responsible for maintaining the functions of almost the entire body. We will take one organ at a time and discuss the research available to help you understand why vitamin D deficiency is a grave medical problem.

Vitamin D and the Heart

Most people who suffer from cardiovascular diseases have been diagnosed with a vitamin D deficiency. Almost every person whose heart has failed has indicated low levels of Vitamin D. For this reason, vitamin D has been recognized as an independent factor responsible for several heart and blood vessel related diseases.

Studies from a research published recently indicated that women with higher ranges of vitamin D levels were 68% less prone to heart diseases in comparison to women in lower range. In men, the risk was 44% lesser. On the other hand, people who had low levels of Vitamin D showed a 42% increase in the risk of acquiring heart related problems. Almost 49- 64% of them were most likely to get a stroke. It was also observed that the chances of having clogged arteries were doubled in individuals with a lower vitamin D level.

The question is how can one nutrient cause people to become susceptible to some of the deadliest diseases in the world? The answer lies in the amount of vitamin D Receptors present. The entire circulatory system including the heart and the blood vessels have a large concentration of vitamin D receptors. This is a clear indication that for optimum performance, vitamin D is required by our circulatory system.

The function of Vitamin D is to create more protective pathways in signals and reduce the occurrence of harmful pathways. Vitamin D is required to ensure that the collagen buildup in the arteries is controlled. They also control the amount of fibrotic proteins that are retained in the heart. These proteins are responsible for the hardening of the artery walls. As a result the blood flow is regulated, keeping blood pressure under control.

These conclusions about the importance of vitamin D for proper functioning of the heart are supported tremendously by compelling studies that have been conducted on human beings. One popular study showed that regular consumption of Vitamin D supplements reduced the chances of inflammation of the arterial walls which was responsible for artherosclerosis. These supplements were also observed to be extremely useful in improving the circulation of blood. Consequently, the blood pressure was also maintained at a desired level.

One part of the population that is the most susceptible to cardiovascular diseases and hypertension is that of African American teens. With a supply of about 2000 IU of vitamin D per day, the actual level of the blood increased significantly. In addition to that, this group also showed a massive drop in the possibility of aortic stiffness and related cardiovascular diseases.

Another experiment conducted on a similar group showed some astounding results. This group was given about 60000IU of vitamin D per day for 4 months. The observation was that the function of the endothelium improved a great deal. The endothelium is a very thin layer of cells that acts as a wall between the blood and the lymph circulating in our body. This layer of cells is responsible for maintaining the pressure of the blood flowing through our veins at a safe level. As a result, the blood pressure was normalized in the study group. A similar test conducted on people who had survived strokes also revealed that the function of the endothelium was highly improved.

One more extremely interesting study group was that of women who were in their late thirties. All these women were either obese or overweight. This is another group that presents extremely high chances of contracting heart related diseases. When these women were given 1000 IU of vitamin D, the observation was that the amount of good cholesterol produced in the body increased tremendously. As a result, the risk of cardiovascular diseases was lowered while also helping these women lower the amount of body mass within just 4 months.

All these tests prove beyond any doubt that vitamin D is extremely essential for our cardiovascular system to function properly. One of the most important functions of vitamin D is the reduction of the hardening of the arterial walls. This is a serious condition that can lead to peripheral arterial disease. When the arteries become hard and narrow, the amount of blood reaching the far ends of the body becomes less. The parts of the body that are most affected are the legs. When people have reduced levels of Vitamin D in their system, they are most likely to develop this condition. The most harrowing consequence of this condition is the amputation of limbs. Studies have revealed that having enough vitamin D can reduce the risk of amputation in people who already suffer from this disease.

The right dose of Vitamin D is extremely important to maintain cardiovascular health. Of course, we know now that that the functions carried out in the heart by Vitamin D are several. Most of these functions are vital to ensure that there are no additional consequences of having problems related to the heart.

When you are consuming Vitamin D for heart related issues, consulting your doctor is ~~extremely~~ essential. You must only consume the recommended amount which is about 2000 IU each day. This number varies according to your age and also your current medical condition. The important thing to remember here is that if you consume amounts lesser than what is recommended, you will see no difference in the health of your heart.

Vitamin D and Diabetes

There is a strong connection between the insulin levels in our body and the Vitamin D level in our body. Although Vitamin D does not directly influence the production of insulin in the body, it is quite apparent that the cells that produce insulin in our body require Vitamin D to perform at their best.

In a study conducted on people with type I and type II diabetes revealed that the level of Vitamin D was significantly low. Even in people who had normal insulin levels, Vitamin D deficiency created a condition called "pre diabetes" that makes you insulin resistant. If you do not have enough Vitamin D intake, you are 91% more likely to develop this "pre-diabetes" condition. Continued Vitamin D deficiency can lead to a progression to type II diabetes. You are at double the risk of developing diabetes if your Vitamin D consumption is not adequate.

Once again, it is the Vitamin D Receptors that play an important role in the connection between diabetes and Vitamin D. All the insulin producing cells in the pancreas have Vitamin D receptors. Additionally, Vitamin D Receptors are found in the cells of our liver and also in the fat and muscle tissues. All these cells that regulate the level of glucose in the blood require Vitamin D to function properly.

In a study of the white blood cells in diabetic patients, the fat content was exceptionally high. The cells used in this study are called macrophages and are a type of white blood cell. Now, the increased fat content in these cells puts the patient with diabetes at a higher risk of contracting cardiovascular diseases. These cells have a tendency to pathologically uptake fat. However, when they were treated in the lab with additional Vitamin D, this tendency reduced, thus reducing any risk of heart related diseases.

A couple of studies performed on animals as well revealed how Vitamin D can increase or decrease the body's resistance to insulin. In comparison to a healthy control group, diabetic animals did not have as many Vitamin D and insulin receptors in their brain. They also accumulated more body fat that the control group, showed signs of inflammation and even DNA damage. These animals scored low in memory tests and revealed reduced cognitive ability. However, continuous intake of Vitamin D supplements was able to restore all these vital functions to almost normal. Cognition, too, improved quite significantly. This study reveals that while Vitamin D deficiency can throw several bodily functions out of balance, replenishing the amount of Vitamin D is also quite successful in restoring the body to its normal condition.

When fat storage in the liver is increased, a condition called non- alcoholic fatty liver disease is developed. This was observed in diabetic animals that underwent inflammatory changes. This condition became worse when the consumption of Vitamin D was not good enough. In human beings, this inflammatory condition could be reduced significantly by maintaining the Vitamin D intake at 1000 IU per day.

While Vitamin D plays an important role in controlling the body's response to insulin, the most important function of Vitamin D is that it reduces the chances of a progression to Type II diabetes from the pre-diabetes condition. Even in obese adults, it was possible to improve glucose regulation and also improve insulin secretion in the pancreas by providing 2000 IU of Vitamin D each day. Even placebos given for 16 weeks were able to produce the same results. When the body is exposed to glucose for a long period of time, the levels of hemoglobin A1c in the blood increase. Even this level was restored with vitamin D supplements. On the other hand, a control group revealed that the conditions became worse when the vitamin D intake was not adequate.

Vitamin D supplements are not useful only when people are in the pre-diabetic or normal stage. Even in people who have already contracted diabetes, Vitamin D is an important nutrient. By consuming about 1000 IU of Vitamin D per day, people with diabetes showed reduced levels of fasting blood sugar and hemoglobin A1c. Their BMI was more regulated, allowing them to keep maintain their body weight. Insulin resistance was also reduced quite significantly. In a control group, however, all these signs increased as they did not get the required amount of vitamin D.

Cholesterol also plays a major role in diabetes and related conditions. Most diabetic people are asked to watch their diet and bring their cholesterol levels down to a recommended number in order to reduce any chances of heart diseases and other conditions arising from diabetes. Studies show that Vitamin D3 is highly responsible for lowering blood pressure, cholesterol level and, particularly, LDL or bad cholesterol levels in the body. These are the three primary risk factors in diabetic people that can lead to conditions of the kidney and the heart. With active Vitamin D3 treatment, the level of proteins in the urine was also brought under control. Usually, increased protein content in the urine is an indicator of kidney problems.

In most people consuming 1200 IU of Vitamin D each day is not as helpful as consuming 2000 IU of Vitamin D each day. The effect that it has on the body is determined by the amount of Vitamin D that is consumed by. When about 2000 IU is consumed every day, blood sugar can be maintained at a required level. The lipid levels in the blood also drop substantially. Heamoglobin A1c level, which indicates diabetes can also be controlled when Vitamin D supplementation is provided.

The most amazing thing about Vitamin D, in relation to diabetes, is that the condition itself is brought under control.

In addition to that, several other problems related to the heart, liver and even kidneys are kept at bay. Diabetes is one of the most feared diseases in the world because it brings the possibility of several other bodily disorders. With Vitamin D consumption, this fear can definitely be replaced with a hope to control of diabetes and also recover faster.

Vitamin D and the Brain Cells

Any neurodegenerative disease like Parkinson's, Dementia or Alzheimer's disease can be prevented by maintaining Vitamin D at the optimum level in our body. Vitamin D is very useful in protecting our brain cells and ensuring their proper functioning for longer periods of time.

Any decline in the cognitive abilities of an individual increases by almost 60% when the Vitamin D consumption is insufficient. People who do not get optimum levels of Vitamin D are 77% more prone to Alzheimer's diseases. The risk of dementia in these people is also 20 times more. Also, when the level of Vitamin D in the body is higher, the intensity of Parkinson's disease is lowered to a large extent.

Our brain cells are highly dependent on the Vitamin D receptors for their proper functioning. As are result supplementation with Vitamin D has the potential to protect and improve the functioning of these brain cells. Most of our brain function depends upon the quality of our nerve cells as well as the speed of transmissions of signals between these cells. With proper intake of Vitamin D, the differentiation of the nerve cells and their growth improves. The nerve connections improve in "plasticity" leading to better learning and also better memory. Nerve transmission is also facilitated by maintaining a recommended level of Vitamin D in the body. On the other hand, all these functions suffer when we neglect the consumption of Vitamin D. These functions may also fail with prolonged deficiency.

Usually, Alzheimer's disease is caused when the amount a certain protein called amyloid beta increases abnormally in our body. This protein is inflammatory in nature and causes degeneration of the brain cells. Studies have revealed that adding vitamin D to nerve cells extracted from Alzheimer's patients has the ability to clear out the amyloid beta protein from the body. This helps in preventing further deterioration and also allows restoration of cells that are not damaged beyond repair.

Some tests conducted on animals also revealed that amyloid beta plaques are developed lesser when Vitamin D is provided. The inflammation of the brain cells also comes down with proper consumption of Vitamin D. The protective nerve growth factor also increases to facilitate better functioning of the brain cells. Studies conducted on a control group provided opposite results as the condition became worse with prolonged Vitamin D deficiency.

Besides reducing the risk of Alzheimer's and other degenerative diseases, Vitamin D also helps improve cognition in brain cells of normal individuals. An experiment conducted on older lab rats revealed that cognitive functioning actually improves quite significantly. These rats usually do not perform well in their cognitive testing. This is probably because hormones and enzymes that promote inflammation of brain cells were more, in addition to larger amounts of amyloid beta proteins in these animals. However, with just about 21 days of regular Vitamin D supplementation, the production of inflammatory enzymes and hormones was reversed and the amyloid beta proteins were cleared faster. Usually, cognition does suffer as age progresses. Even if it does not lead to severe conditions like Alzheimer's the speed of cognition will reduced with age. Consuming enough vitamin D will help you prevent this cognitive decline.

Another major degenerative age related disease is Parkinson's. This disease is extremely difficult to manage as it affects the entire nervous system. It reduces an individual's ability to perform simple daily functions such as walking and eating in severe conditions. The advantage of providing Vitamin D supplementation to the elderly is that with improved cognition, their chances of falling reduces to a large extent. They are also able to balance themselves better. These are the biggest problems faced by patients with Parkinson's disease. Consuming about 1200 IU of Vitamin D3 per day is good enough to prevent further deterioration in individuals with Parkinson's disease. When consumed over 12 months continuously, these supplements are actually capable of controlling the intensity of Parkinson's in these patients. Of course, the type of Vitamin D Receptors may vary from one individual to another. Consequently, the effect of Vitamin D might be greater or lesser.

The conclusion that these tests provide is that Vitamin D, Vitamin D3 in particular, has the ability to protect the cells in our brain. The functioning of our neurons and the cells in our brain is improved to promote longevity and good health.

Vitamin D and Autoimmune Diseases

It is important to maintain a balance in our immune system in order to make it efficient against microorganisms that may attack and invade our body. Studies have shown that the cells in our immune system, too, have high levels of Vitamin D Receptors. Therefore, the modulation of the immune system requires a continuous supply of Vitamin D. Only when the immune system receives a certain amount of Vitamin D does it become ready to assume the "attack mode" when any outside threat is detected. It must also switch to the "clean up" mode when the threat is over. This modulation is extremely important to ensure that the tissues in our body are not damaged by the response of the immune system.

Vitamin D is definitely necessary to help the immune system switch from one mode to another. It has another important role to play with respect to the immune system. Sometimes when this modulation falls out of balance, the immune system reacts to normal tissues and cells as if they are a threat. This type of reaction can be against a single tissue or organ or can also attack several organs at one given time. The diseases arising out of this abnormal response of the immune system are called auto immune diseases.

The role of Vitamin D in our body becomes important to manage the onset and also the progression of these diseases. Some common auto immune diseases that Vitamin D is effective against are- lupus, Type I diabetes, rheumatoid arthritis and also multiple sclerosis.

According to research, restoring the level of Vitamin D in the body helps improve the production of T cells in the Body.

These T- cells are responsible for the proper functioning of the immune system. It is possible to restore the immune system from its overactive state to its normal state by increasing the production of these T-cells.

By increasing the amount of Vitamin D in the Body, it is also possible to acquire certain benefits that are disease specific. For instance:

- In patients suffering from lupus or rheumatoid arthritis, the activity of the disease is decreased.
- In case off Type I diabetes, the onset of the condition itself can be prevented with proper consumption of Vitamin D. The pancreatic cells that are responsible for the production of insulin are protected in order to regulate the level of insulin in the body.
- In several studies conducted on animals, the development of multiple sclerosis is also reduced. With humans, the risk of onset of multiple sclerosis is reduced by almost 40%.

So you see, sometimes our body needs to be protected from itself. If we are not alert enough, a slight imbalance of nutrients in the body can lead to our body fighting against itself. So, it is important that we all maintain a balanced diet in the real sense. The consumption of Vitamin D in particular should never be ignored. With just a few minutes out in the sun, think of the number of diseases that can be controlled and even prevented!

Vitamin D and Cancer

No matter how much we progress in terms of medical technology and research, the idea of cancer is extremely intimidating. Although this is a genetic disease that has no real preventive measure, it is possible to reduce the risk of several types of cancers by increasing the level of Vitamin D in the body. Studies have revealed that restoring Vitamin D is very important in blocking the manifestation of cancer.

Low levels of Vitamin D in the body can, in fact, increase your chances of developing cancerous cells within the body. Studies revealed that people who had higher levels of Vitamin D are almost 150% less likely to develop cancer in comparison to people with lower levels of Vitamin D.

There are several pathways that are created in our body to signal the growth of tumors and also inflammation of cells. There are also certain pathways that guide the surveillance of our immune system for cancer. All these pathways are controlled by Vitamin D Receptors that are found in cells. In the skin cells, prostate cells, colon cells and the breast cells, the role of these Vitamin D Receptors against cancer is the highest. We all know that these tissues are also most prone to cancer in comparison to the rest of our body.

In cells that are cancerous, the level of Vitamin D Receptors is extremely low. As a result, these cells are not properly regulated and tend to multiply uncontrollably. That is how they turn into tumors. When cancer cell cultures in labs were treated with Vitamin D, several important functions were regulated. The proliferation of the tumor cells reduced, inflammation in the cells was suppressed and the chances of tumor cell death or apostasies increased. These factors are responsible for helping our body fight against cancer.

The three types of cancers that are benefitted the most from an increase in the level of Vitamin D in the body are that of the breast, colon and prostate.

Vitamin D and Breast Cancer

A series of tests were conducted on animals in which breast cancer was induced. The observations revealed that the size of the tumor, the number of tumors and also the incidence of tumors was reduced with Vitamin D supplementation. The effect was increased when Vitamin D was mixed with DHA and EPA derived from fish oil.

Estrogen dependent breast cancer benefitted greatly with active Vitamin D3 consumption. Estrogen has the ability to promote the growth of tumors in the breast tissue. By restoring the level of Vitamin D3, it became possible to suppress enzymes that were responsible for the production of estrogen. As a result the alpha form of estrogen that is responsible for promoting malignant tumors was also reduced.

A study conducted as part of a Women's Health initiative revealed that even low doses of vitamin D when combined with calcium supplements had the ability to reduce the chances of breast cancer in women by almost 20% in comparison to a control group.

Vitamin D and Prostate Cancer

Prostate cancer responds very strongly to Vitamin D supplementation, according to a series of tests conducted on men who were given 4000 IU of Vitamin D each day for one entire year. Individuals who had tumor positive biopsies showed an improvement in the condition and a reduction in these biopsies. The Gleason tumor score, which is a major concern in prostate cancer also reduced to a large extent. In about 11% of these individuals, progression of cancer was not observed. Malignancy in prostate cancer is slow- growing.

Therefore, it is a great idea to consume Vitamin D as a preventive measure.

Vitamin D and Colon Cancer

Chronic inflammation is responsible for the progression to malignancy in rectum and colon cancer. The inflammatory markers in patients with colorectal adenoma reduced by 77% when they were given 800 IU of Vitamin D every day. This is an important step towards preventing the progression of cancer in the colon and rectum. When a similar group was given about 800 IU of vitamin D3 each day, the levels of tumor suppressors increased significantly. In' addition to that, the levels of tumor promoters were also reduced significantly allowing the cells to restore themselves to normalcy.

Vitamin D is one nutrient that has several positive effects on our body. From regulating cell division to moderating the immune system, it is one nutrient that plays an important role. So, it goes beyond doubt that Vitamin D is, indeed, a miracle nutrient.

Chapter 8: The Effects of Vitamin D Deficiency

We have established that vitamin D is responsible for the proper functioning of almost all organs in our body. Still, the lack of knowledge about Vitamin D supplementation has led to severe vitamin D deficiency across the globe. Like any other nutrient, the decrease in Vitamin D levels in our bodies leads to several problems. The most common diseases that are associated with vitamin D deficiency are related to the bone. This is because the major role of Vitamin D is in the absorption of calcium and Phosphorous. The most common Vitamin D deficiency induced diseases are:

Rickets

Rickets is a condition that is almost synonymous with vitamin D deficiency. It is the study of this disease that led to the discovery of vitamin D itself. Rickets leads to improper development of the bones. The bones developed as a result of rickets are usually soft and weak. Growth is stunted and there are also skeletal deformities in severe cases. One of the most common sights in children with rickets is bow shaped legs. These legs are curved outwards leading to difficulty in walking and performing proper movements in the limbs.

Rickets is mostly observed in children between the ages of 6 to 24 months. The skeletal system in children is still in the stage of development. It is necessary for several bones to fuse and even grow to create a proper skeletal framework. Any nutritional problem in this age can lead to reduced calcium and phosphorous absorption. As a result the bones are weak, under developed and even deformed in some cases. It is possible that rickets is inherited genetically in some individuals.

The geographical location of individuals also plays an important role in the possibility of developing rickets. Children who live in areas with lesser sunlight are more likely to have bone deformities and also rickets.

Signs and Symptoms of Rickets

Visible bone deformity is common in children with rickets. However, the common signs and symptoms include:
- Persistent pain and tenderness in the bones. The most affected regions are the spine, pelvis, legs and arms.
- Tooth formation is significantly delayed. There may be deformity in the dental structure and also holes and abscesses in the enamel.

- Growth is impaired and is usually stunted in children who suffer from rickets. As a result their stature is quite short.
- Muscle cramps are often as the bones required for them to attach themselves to are deformed.
- Since the bones are brittle, the chances of fractures are also higher.
- Several skeletal deformities like bumps on the ribcage, bowlegs, oddly shaped skull, protruding sternum and even a curved spine may be observed in children with rickets.

Diagnosis and Treatment

A simple physical examination is good enough to determine if the child is suffering from rickets or not. There are also obvious signs like pain in the bone and tenderness in the joints. To confirm the condition, a blood test to determine the level of calcium or phosphorus might be necessary. Doctors may also take a look at the structure and the formation of the bones with the help of X-rays and scans to confirm the condition. In some cases a bone biopsy might be required. The bone fluid is extracted and observed to draw final conclusions in a diagnosis.

Replacing the missing nutrient in the body is the best way to treat rickets. This can be done through supplements and also reliable food sources like fish and milk. Vitamin D deficiency will also require an individual to spend more time in the sun to allow the body to synthesize Vitamin D naturally.

Osteomalacia

This is one of the most severe consequences of vitamin D deficiency. When the amount of Vitamin D available to the body is inadequate, the ability of the bones to absorb calcium and phosphorous reduces to a large extent. This hinders the building process of the bones and results in soft and brittle bones. This is a formative disease that is usually due to the unavailability of calcium and phosphorous for the bones to absorb for proper structure and strength.

There are several indirect factors that contribute to the occurrence of osteomalacia in an individual. In case of any surgical procedure that has resulted in the removal of the small intestine, the absorption of Vitamin D is restricted. This further restricts the assimilation of Calcium in the body, causing improper formation of the bones. Even diseases like celiac disease or cancer that interfere with the ability of the body to absorb nutrients can lead to osteomalacia. Liver and

Kidney disorders that affect Vitamin D metabolism may also lead to Osteomalacia.

Signs and Symptoms

The most common sign of osteomalacia is brittle bones that tend to fracture very easily. Even with a small fall, it is possible for severe fractures to occur. This is a matter of concern as osteomalacia usually occurs in children.

Our bones and muscles work hand in hand. Some weakness in one of them leads to weakness in the other. As a result, people with osteomalacia will experience muscle weakness as well. This is because the area where the muscle is attached to the bone is affected. This leads to inability to perform a complete range of motion in that area. Most common problems are difficulty in walking and also an improper gait.

Pain in the joints is also common. The area where the individual will experience maximum pain is the hip. The nature of the pain is quite dully and achy. This pain will radiate to the legs, lower back and even the ribs in extreme conditions.

Since osteomalacia is related to reduced calcium levels in the body, there are chances of experiencing irregular heartbeats.

Numbness in the arms and legs and around the mouth is also a common symptom.

Diagnosis and Treatment

Usually, blood tests are recommended to test the level of vitamin D in the body. The calcium and phosphorus levels also need to be determined for conclusive diagnosis. In case there are high levels of alkaline phospatase isozymes, osteomalacia is suspected. The level of parathyroid hormone is also useful in detecting the possibility of osteomalacia. If the level of this hormone is high, the chances of vitamin D deficiency are also high.

Treatment of Osteomalacia is possible through oral Vitamin D supplements. It is necessary for patients to restore the vitamin D level in the body at an earlier stage. In severe cases, vitamin D is also administered intravenously.

Osteoporosis

The name osteoporosis is derived from a Latin word which translates to porous bones. This condition usually arises when the space inside the bone increases abnormally. Usually, inside the bone, there are tiny spaces that resemble a honeycomb. In case of osteoporosis, these spaces increase reducing the density and strength of the bones. The exterior of the bone also becomes weaker with osteoporosis.

This condition is very severe since the risk of fractures is very high. A person may break a bone even while standing or walking. Research by the National Institute of Health revealed that almost 40 million people are affected by osteoporosis globally.

Unlike osteomalacia that affects the bones in the formative years, osteoporosis causes brittleness and deformity of the bones after it has been completely formed. As a result, this is a degenerative disease that progresses with age. Usually, people who are about 30 years old witness the onset of this condition. The density of the bone falls rapidly without replacing the necessary nutrients at the same rate. In women, this condition usually occurs around their onset of menopause.

Osteoporosis is most likely to develop in individuals who are older in age, who have very poor nutrition, who have a line of osteoporosis in their family history, who smoke and also perform very little physical activity.

Symptoms of Osteoporosis

The problem with osteoporosis is that there is absolutely no warning sign or symptom in the initial stages. In many cases, people do not even know that they have osteoporosis till they have a fracture. Fractures in the spine are common with people who have osteoporosis. Another common occurrence as osteoporosis progresses is the bending of the spine and also a sudden loss of height.

Diagnosis and Treatment

The bone density can be scanned to determine the possibility of osteoporosis. A painless scan called the dual ray X-ray absorptiometry is performed to check the bone density. The density of the bones in the spine, hips and wrist are checked first as these areas are most likely to develop osteoporosis. Even if a person is at a risk of developing osteoporosis, this scan may be performed. Usually a bone density scan is conducted in case of a fracture to check if the cause for the fracture is osteoporosis.

There are several ways to treat osteoporosis. Usually bio-phosponate drugs are recommended for the treatment of osteoporosis. These medicines prevent any reduction of bone mass. They may be administered orally or even intravenously.

Hormone treatments like testosterone treatments in men and estrogen treatments in women can play a very important role in reducing the loss of bone mass. There are also alternative medications like Vitamin D supplements that can help control the condition. The only sad part about osteoporosis is that preventive measures are very few. Since the most common causal factors are genetic or gender related, preventive care is not an option. However, pain management and rehabilitation can easy the condition largely.

Osteoarthritis

Osteoarthritis is a form of arthritis that is characterized by the breakdown of the cartilages in the joints of the bones. In comparison to the various forms of arthritis, osteoarthritis is most common as it affects close to 25 million people in the US alone. This condition is usually age dependent. In men, it is most likely to appear before they turn 45 while in women, it occurs after the age of 55. It is also known as degenerative arthritis or degenerative bone disease as it is age dependent.

As the condition progresses, there are chances of complete loss of this cartilage in the joints.

The role of the cartilage between the joints is to provide some cushioning during movement and also heavy impact on the joints. Usually, osteoarthritis is prominent in the joints of the hands, feet, hips, knees and also the spine. These joints are used the most or bear the maximum amount of weight in comparison to other joints in the body.

Signs and symptoms

There are several types of arthritis and osteoarthritis is one of them. Most forms of arthritis spread to several areas in the body and may also affect the whole body with progression of the condition. In case of osteoarthritis, however, a single joint is affected.

The common symptom of osteoarthritis is the inflammation of the joints resulting in extreme pain in the affected area. Sometimes, the affected joint will seem warm for prolonged periods of time. Additionally, a creaking sound may also be heard when you try to move the joint. When the condition progresses, the friction between the bones also increases causing excruciating pain and reduced range of motion. This is because the cartilage between the bones is lost completely.

The level of pain experienced varies from one person to another. Sometimes, a person may feel very little pain even when X-rays reveal extreme degeneration of the bones. On the other hand, some of them might experience a lot of pain even at the onset of osteoarthritis. The pain depends on several factors like the area affected and also nutrition.

Diagnosis and Treatment

Osteoarthritis is usually diagnosed with the help of X-rays. In severe conditions, the bone fluid may be extracted to understand the extent of damage. Arthroscopy is also a recommended method for diagnosis of Osteoarthritis.

Exercise is one of the best ways to treat this condition. Also, intake of Vitamin D supplements can control the condition and prevent further damage.

Other Vitamin D Deficiency Diseases

As we have learned from the earlier chapter, Vitamin D is necessary for the proper functioning of several parts of our body. Therefore, it is obvious that Vitamin D deficiency will affect several organs besides the bones. Some of the most common problems occurring from vitamin D deficiency in the body include:

- Lack of blood pressure regulation in people who are already suffering from hypertension.
- Increased incidence of type II diabetes.
- Increase chances of contracting cardiovascular diseases.

- Increased severity in cardiovascular diseases, diabetes and also hypertension.

- Increased inflammation in cells due to reduced moderation of inflammation markers.

- Increased susceptibility to allergies in adolescents and children. A test conducted on about 6000 individuals revealed that sensitization to allergies was greater in children and adolescents whose vitamin D level was lower than 15 ng/ml. This is probably because of the close association between Vitamin D and the proper functioning of the immune system.

- The occurrence of dental cavities also increased with reduced levels of Vitamin D. This is possibly associated with the lack of proper calcium absorption. It was observed that proper vitamin D supplementation reduced the occurrence of cavities in the teeth by almost 47%

- Increased chances of depression. Our brain cells consist of several vitamin D receptors that are responsible for the occurrence and the intensity of depression. Since Vitamin D is also associated with several other brain processes, its association with depression and related psychological disorders is not really shocking.

- Increase in Erectile Dysfunction: Although there is no clear association between erectile dysfunction and vitamin D, it has been observed that vitamin D supplementation can lead to reduced ED. This is possibly because Vitamin D is related to cardiovascular diseases. Most men who suffer from erectile dysfunction are likely to have cardiovascular diseases.

- Reduced cholesterol regulation. One of the primary methods of synthesizing vitamin D in the body is by breaking down cholesterol derivatives. So, reduced exposure to sunlight is capable of increasing the cholesterol levels in the body.

While many of the problems mentioned above are affected by vitamin D deficiency at a very secondary level, it is wrong to assume that the incidence and intensity of these conditions is entirely independent of the Vitamin D level in our body. While we usually look at the primary causal factors for several disorders, the actual solution may lie in the revision of our diet and nutrition. Most disorders are closely related to lack of nutrition. By keeping an eye on the Vitamin D intake alone, it is possible to get rid of so many commonly occurring disorders.

Chapter 9: What Causes Vitamin D Deficiency?

The most common cause for vitamin D deficiency is associated with our lack of proper nutrition. However, unknown to most people, vitamin D deficiency goes way beyond nutritional causes. This is another important reason why vitamin D deficiency is a serious epidemic. Nobody knows what the real causes for vitamin D deficiency are. Sometimes, just taking necessary amounts of supplements cannot solve the issue of vitamin D Deficiency. The other contributing factors to this global epidemic are:

Reduced exposure to Sunlight

One of the biggest myths of our time is that exposure to sunlight causes skin cancer. There is no doubt that the harmful UV rays of the sun might have damaging effects on the skin. However, what nobody really discusses is the possibility of vitamin D deficiency with reduced exposure to the sun.

What are causes reduced exposure to the sun? First, we all spend several hours indoors thanks to our lifestyles. Second, we all believe in using sunscreen every time we step out into the sun. The idea is to prevent damage to the skin cells.

However, here is some information that might make you think twice about using sunscreen the next time. Sunscreen with SPF 30 has the ability to reduce the synthesis of vitamin D in the skin by almost 95%!

There are several factors like the season, your geographical location and also the time of the day that determine the efficiency of Vitamin D synthesis in your body. Also, the amount of exposure that you get is also important in determining the amount of vitamin D that is produced in the body. Logically, it may seem like staying in the sun for long hours will result in better production of Vitamin D. However, the truth is actually quite contrary.

As we have discussed before, the process of Vitamin D synthesis in our body is far more complex than just a few minutes in the sun. There are several chemical reactions that take place in order to create the required amount of Vitamin D in the body. These reactions are not facilitated by prolonged exposure to the sun. Instead, short periods of exposure to the sun will help improve the production of Vitamin D in the body. Additionally, you also do not put your skin at the risk of damage or burning by limiting the time that you spend in the sun. For most people, spending about 15 minutes in the sun can work wonders.

Dark Skin

The color of our skin is dependent on a pigment known as melanin. The lesser the melanin in our body, the lighter is the skin. The primary function of the melanin in our skin is to absorb the UV rays from the sun. This reduces the formation of vitamin D in the skin as the required amount of UV rays is not received. Therefore, people who have darker skin will find it harder to synthesize Vitamin D in their body. In comparison to lighter people, darker people will require close to five time more exposure to sunlight to produce the amount of Vitamin D required by the body. Comparisons of vitamin D levels in lighter and darker people in the same geographical location revealed that darker people need more sunlight to make vitamin D.

Obesity

Studies have revealed that the Body Mass Index plays a very vital role in maintaining the Vitamin D levels in the body. One such study was conducted on 2000 overweight and obese individuals. The observations revealed that people with a Body Mass Index above 40 showed 18% less levels of vitamin D in their serum in comparison to individuals who had BMI lower than 40.

Another study conducted exclusively on 154 obese individuals and 148 non obese individuals revealed that the vitamin D level in the obese individuals was 23% lesser that the non obese individuals. One of the most common reasons for the lower levels of vitamin D is the necessity of higher vitamin D distribution in obese individuals. Even with adequate exposure to the sun, the chances of maintaining a balance between the amount of Vitamin D required by the body and the amount of Vitamin D synthesized in the body in never met.

A study conducted on obese individuals after exposure to sunlight revealed that they still exhibited 57% less vitamin D in comparison to individuals who were not obese. Although there is no clear evidence to suggest why obesity causes reduced levels of Vitamin D, the truth is that the two go hand in hand. Therefore, it is advisable for obese people to consult their doctors and consume necessary supplements.

There are several other reasons why Vitamin D level in the body can be low. One of the causal factors is mal-absorption. In individuals who suffer from diseases like celiac disease and Crohn's disease and also in people who have undergone surgeries, a reduction in the Vitamin D level is observed. In certain instances where the small intestine has been surgically removed, there are chances of reduced vitamin D absorption. Individuals who suffer from these conditions are unable to take in the amount of fat soluble vitamin D that their body requires.

If you are currently taking any medication, there are chances that your ability to synthesize and absorb Vitamin D will reduce. There are several antifungal medicines, glucocorticoids, anti-convulsion medicines and also AIDS/HIV medicines that can result in reduced levels of vitamin D in the body.

People who suffer from conditions like chronic kidney disease, hyperpaprathyroidism and also lymphoma will be unable to produce and absorb Vitamin D efficiently.

In any case, it is a good idea to have your vitamin D levels tested on a regular basis just to be sure. It is very difficult for several people to get the necessary amount of Vitamin D from fortified foods and also exposure to sunlight. Depending upon your current medical condition, the supplements that you require to restore the level of vitamin D in your body can be very different. For several individuals, even getting the minimum recommended level of vitamin D can be a challenge owing to several physical conditions.

Chapter 10: Population Groups Prone to Vitamin D Deficiency

There are certain sections of the population that require special care to maintain the vitamin D levels in their body. These sections of the population include:

Infants who are being breastfed

Children who are being breast fed have human milk as the only source of nutrition. The level of vitamin D is lesser than 25 IU per liter making human milk an inadequate source. The amount of vitamin D that is found in breast milk is closely related to the amount of Vitamin D that is present in the mother's body. Studies show that mothers who take high doses of Vitamin D supplements are likely to have a larger level of Vitamin D in the milk.

In a review of a report made on nutritional rickets, several cases indicated that this condition occurred mostly in breast fed African American children. Another Canadian research revealed that the incidence of rickets in the study group was quite high. Almost all cases of rickets in this study, too, indicated breast feeding. Infants are also kept away from sunlight as their skin is extremely sensitive. Even when they are out in the sun, it is necessary for them to wear ample protective clothing. It is recommended by the AAS that infants who are exclusively breastfed must be given at least 400 IU of vitamin D supplements per day to reduce the incidence of conditions like rickets.

The Elderly

Older people are more likely to develop vitamin D deficiency for several reasons. One important reason is that the skin loses its ability to synthesize vitamin D efficiently. They also spend a lot of time indoors because of which the amount of sun exposure required to produce vitamin D is not available. This is why several elders are at the risk of hip and pelvic fractures. Due to the reduction in the vitamin D level, the amount of calcium absorbed falls as well. Most elders in the USA have less than 12ng/ml of vitamin D in their serum.

People with fat mal-absorption

It is a known fact that Vitamin D is a fat soluble vitamin. The ability of the intestines to absorb dietary fats influences the ability of Vitamin D absorption. In case an individual is unable to absorb dietary fats, he may require vitamin D supplementation. There are several conditions that reduce the body's ability to absorb fat. These conditions include Celic disease, liver disorders and even fibrosis. Some people may also be under a diet that requires them to reduce the intake of foods that contain adequate dietary fats.

If you are under a diet that restricts the consumption of Vitamin D rich foods, there may be a drop in the level of Vitamin D in your body. Even women who wear long garments and cover their head do not get enough sunlight to synthesize vitamin D in the body. Of course the increased use of sunscreen is a matter of primary concern. In addition to all this spending too much time indoors and also not getting the right kind of nutrition will lead to Vitamin D deficiency eventually.

Chapter 11: Vitamin D Deficiency and Geographical Location

Since the synthesis of Vitamin D in our body depends upon the amount of sunlight that we receive, it is quite obvious that the geographical location of makes a great difference. As we know, the amount of sunlight received in different parts of the globe and the type of sunlight received are extremely different. As a result, the amount of sunlight required by each person must also vary.

Health experts believe that it is not possible to provide a universal recommendation for vitamin D supplementation. Depending upon the area that a person lives in, his or her chances of acquiring vitamin D deficiency will also vary. For instance, men from the African American race are more likely to suffer from Vitamin D deficiency when they live in areas with low sunlight. On the other hand, European men living in the same area are not as prone to vitamin D deficiency. This report is based on a study that was recently conducted in a certain area in Chicago.

A test conducted in about 492 men in the age group of 40-79 years to study the level of vitamin D in their body. These men lived in Chicago Illinois. It was observed that men form an African American descent had 93% vitamin D deficiency. On the other hand, European men in the same test group had just 69.5% vitamin D deficiency.

This study made it quite obvious that having a universal recommendation for vitamin D supplementation is extremely futile. A study conducted on several other groups also revealed that the amount of Vitamin D was quite different in men who had higher BMI. This study also shows clearly that it is not just the amount of sunlight received but also the type of skin and the current physical condition of an individual that is responsible for the amount of Vitamin D in his body.

Three Types of Radiation

The basis of the synthesis of Vitamin D in the body is that the exposure of certain cholesterol derivatives to UV rays from the sun results in the synthesis of Vitamin D. The sun produces several types of radiations. The three most common ones that we come in contact with on a regular basis are: UVA, UVB and UVC. Out of these three types of UV radiations, UVB is most effective is producing Vitamin D in our skin. With UVA, there are chances of aging and wrinkles with constant exposure. UVC rays are extremely dangerous as they have the ability to cause sunburns.

The type of radiation received in your area plays an important role in the amount of time that you can spend in the sun. Consequently, the amount of Vitamin D produced will also vary. As a result, geographical location plays a very important role in the synthesis of Vitamin D. Even the season and the time of the day will determine the effects the amount of Vitamin D that is synthesized in the body.

Geography and the Ability to Make Vitamin D

It is true that the amount of vitamin D in the body depends upon the geographical location of an individual. However, there is no substantial evidence to support this statement. It is true that the UV rays of the sun trigger the production of Vitamin D in the body. In areas located at higher altitudes, the UVB radiation received from the sun is low. As a result, the amount of Vitamin D produced by these individuals is low. On the other hand, people living closer to the equator have a higher level of Vitamin D.

Some studies conducted in several areas across the globe point quite strongly to the fact that people living in areas with low levels of sunlight are likely to suffer from related deficiency diseases. For instance, a child living in Finland is 400 times more likely to develop conditions related to reduced Vitamin D levels. These diseases include multiple sclerosis, type 1diabetes and also solon cancer. The question that arose here was if it was only reduced exposure to sunlight that created these problems or was it the reduction in Vitamin D levels altogether?

Several theories and hypotheses about Vitamin D and the related diseases are associated with studies that compare solar radiations in these areas. There have been several descriptive geographical studies that have been conducted to understand the relationship between the Vitamin D production and the geographical location of individuals. So far, the studies have only indicated that the risk for certain diseases is related to the geographical location of the individual.

However, studies that were conducted in further detail made the association between Vitamin D Deficiency related diseases and geographical location weaker. It was observed that certain lifestyle changes could contribute significantly towards the reduction of the intensity of diseases. Colon cancer for instance could be reduced in areas with lower sunlight by just increasing the consumption of fiber. There were several other ecological studies that revealed that the level of Vitamin D alone could not determine the possibility of certain diseases in a given geographical location.

What is interesting to note is that the amount of exposure that you require in the sun to synthesize Vitamin D deferens form one area to another. For instance, in Brisbane, Australia, the amount of sunlight exposure required is about 6-7 minutes in summer and about 30 minutes in winter. On the other hand the amount of exposure to sunlight required in Hobart is about 9 minutes in summer and about 50 minutes in winter. Although these areas are not too far from each other, the type of sunrays received is significantly different. As a result the time of exposure varies.

It is interesting to learn more about geography and Vitamin D as the research always shows varying results. In my research, the revelation was that the diseases caused may not depend upon the geographical location but the amount of sunlight that you require does vary.

Chapter 12: Best Sources of Vitamin D

The synthesis of Vitamin D in our body is one of the primary sources of vitamin D in our body. Therefore the primary source of Vitamin D in our body is sun exposure. It is possible for most people to meet the minimum requirement of vitamin D in their body by exposure to sunlight. Ultraviolet radiation which is of a wavelength between 290 and 320 nanometers has the ability to penetrate through our skin. When the light reaches our skin a series of photochemical reactions begin. The first set of these reactions involve the conversion of 7-dehydrocholesterol to the most active form of Vitamin D-Vitamin D3. There are several factors that determine the efficiency of sun exposure in providing the amount of sunlight required by our body. These factors include the length of the day, the time of the day, the presence of smog or fog and also cloud cover. There are several factors that are intrinsic as well. These factors include the melanin deposit of our skin, age and the current physical condition of our body. Besides these factors, the use of sunscreen can also affect the amount of Vitamin D produced to a large extent. Of course, as we discussed before, there is no consistency in the pattern of Vitamin D production with a change in geographical location. There are several opportunities available for the body to synthesize vitamin D in the absence of sunlight. Sometimes,

Vitamin D is also stored in the liver and in the fat cells for utilization at a later stage.

In case of complete cloud cover, the amount of UV rays that reach us reduce by almost 50%. It is also true that UV rays cannot penetrate through glass. So exposure to sunlight through the window will actually do your body no good. It is also possible for our skin to synthesize vitamin D when there is a layer of sunscreen on the skin. Of course, the amount of Vitamin D produced is lesser and most health practitioners recommend exposure of the skin without any protection to achieve best results.

Because of these several factors that determine the amount of sunlight required, it is impossible to provide a perfect recommendation chart for the amount of sunlight that you must expose your ski to every single day. On an average, studies indicate that any amount of exposure from 5- 30 minutes between 10 AM in the Morning and 3 PM in the afternoon can be of great use to the skin in the production of Vitamin D. Some people also prefer to use commercial tanning beds to get their dose of UV rays. These beds are capable of producing 2-6% of UVB rays. However, it is best recommended that you rely upon natural sources to get your daily dose of proteins.

Food

The options available with respect to food sources of Vitamin D are not many. In the most natural form, fatty fish like mackerel, tuna and salmon contain high levels of Vitamin D. Fish liver oil is considered the best and the most reliable source of Vitamin D. You can also find traces of vitamin D in beef liver, egg yolks and cheese. In all these natural sources, vitamin D is available in the form of Vitamin D3. Therefore, these foods are highly recommended as they give us a direct source of the most active biological form of Vitamin D3. It is also possible to obtain vitamin D from mushrooms that have been subjected to UV radiation. These mushrooms contain high levels of vitamin D2 and are a preferred source of nutrition among vegans and vegetarians.

There are several fortified foods out there in the market to provide us with the necessary amounts of vitamin D. Most of the milk supply in the United States consists of 100IU of vitamin D per cup. In countries like Canada, about 35- 40IU of Vitamin D is available per cup. Fortifying foods with Vitamin D became a common practice after a program was implemented in the USA to prevent rickets in children. By the 1930s, rickets had become a major health concern and had to be eradicated. As a result, fortified foods were introduced into the market. Today several dairy products including milk and cheese contain Vitamin D. Even fun foods like ice creams come with Vitamin D. Several juice brands also fortify their products to make them more nutritious.

Supplements

As I had mentioned before, dietary supplements are available in two forms- Vitamin D2 supplements and Vitamin D3 supplements. The difference between these two forms of supplements is that while D2 is derived from plant sources, D3 is derived from animal sources. The nutritional doses and the price of both these supplements are just the same. However, higher doses of Vitamin D2 supplements are less potent in comparison to Vitamin D3 supplements.

It is recommended that all children who are being breast fed must consume necessary supplements. Even adults who do not get adequate exposure to sunlight can consider Vitamin Supplements as a favorable nutrition option. For infants supplementation of Vitamin D must happen only through fortified foods like milk. The recommended intake of these supplements is as per the recommendation of your doctor.

No matter what source of Vitamin D you choose, the good news is that replenishing the amount of Vitamin D in your body is quite simple. All you need to do is be aware of the foods that you are consuming. You can also ask a nutritionist's advice on the amount of Vitamin D that your body requires each day. The amount of Vitamin D in the several sources can also be calculated to understand which one is most beneficial to you and your requirements. Remember that an overdose of Vitamin D can also induce toxicity in the body.

Chapter 12: Diagnosis of Vitamin D Deficiency

Diagnosis of vitamin D deficiency is extremely simple. All you need to undergo is a simple blood test. It is possible to check the levels of various other hormones and nutrients in the body to confirm if you have a vitamin D deficiency or not. It is not very simple, however, to determine the optimal level of vitamin D in your body. The term optimal level of Vitamin D itself is shrouded in controversy as the levels can vary largely from one individual to another. In order to check your blood for Vitamin D deficiency, a certain factor known as 25 (OH) D levels is checked. Depending upon the level of this factor, there are certain guidelines of the Institute of Medical Health that can help determine if an individual has a deficiency or not.

Here are regular parameters that are used to determine if you do have a deficiency of Vitamin D or not.

If the level of 25(OH)D is below 12 ng/ml, the individual is said to have a deficiency.
Any level between 12-50 ng/ml is considered inadequate
Levels of 25(OH) D between 25- 50 ng/ml is considered adequate.
Any level above 50 ng/ ml is considered excessive.

It is believed widely that the ideal amount of Vitamin D3 in the body should be about 30 ng/ml for optimal body functioning. However, a national survey conducted in the year 2004 revealed that the amount of Vitamin D required is actually about 24 ng/ml. Therefore the parameters also increased by 2-6%.

It is sad that there is no way to determine the actual level of Vitamin D that your body requires to function at its best. With the parameters changing on a regular basis, it has also become difficult to maintain global awareness about the right amount of Vitamin D required by the body. As a result, it the deficiency of vitamin D has also become an epidemic.

It is important for each one of us to gain more insight into this subject in order to be able to provide the body with the nutrition that it requires. It is possible for us to determine, on an individual level, the amount of vitamin D that is necessary. You can also watch out for obvious signs in the body that will tell you if you need to undergo treatment for a possible deficiency of Vitamin D.

How to Improve Vitamin D intake?

Now that we have established the Vitamin D intake required for our body, it is important to learn how you can replenish the levels of vitamin D. There are several approved techniques that you can opt for after consulting your doctor. Some such techniques are:

Injections

You can get vitamin D injections that will last for several months. Even a small injection is capable of lasting up to 6 months. This is one of the most effective and convenient treatment methods. This treatment method is perfect for you if you do not like taking tablets. Even if you have the tendency of forgetting these tablets, you can opt for injections.

High Dose liquids and tablets

Depending upon your current vitamin D deficiency level, the strength of your tablet or liquid will change. In case you are suffering from a high level of vitamin D deficiency, it is recommended that you consume high dose tablets or powders. These high dose supplements will allow you to improve your situation faster. High doses are recommended for growing children.

Standard dose liquids, tablets and Powders

In order to maintain the balance of vitamin D in your body on a regular basis, it is important for you to take standard dose supplements. Although the action of these supplements can be quite slow, you can take them as preventive measures.

The most important thing in vitamin D deficiency treatment is the maintenance therapy. After the level of vitamin D has been restored in your body, you must make sure your body undergoes enough maintenance in order to prevent a decline in the level of Vitamin D in the future. It is important to continue milder doses of vitamin D supplements in order to have long term benefits.

Preventive Measures against Vitamin D Deficiency

In case you are not suffering from any apparent deficiency of vitamin D in your body, you may take preventive measures. According to the Chief Medical Officers of the United Kingdom, the following methods work well in preventing Vitamin D deficiency:

- Pregnant and breast feeding women should consume at least 10 mg of Vitamin D every day.
- Infants and children up to 5 years of age should be given vitamin drops every day. In case the child is feeding on formula, the amount of Vitamin D supplement required is lesser.
- People who are 65 years of age or older, must try and get as much sunshine as possible in order to maintain their vitamin D levels.

No matter what supplement you take or treatment method you choose, make sure you consult a doctor. In case you have conditions like liver and kidney diseases, the methods are more specific and strategic.

Chapter 15: What Happens with Excess Vitamin D?

Is it possible to get too much of a good thing? Apparently it is! While proper consumption of Vitamin D has several benefits, there is also a chance that you are overdoing it. Sometimes, people get too worked up about a possible deficiency and begin to give their body a lot more than it requires.

It is true that any nutrient that exceeds the recommended amount in the body will lead to poisoning. When the level of Vitamin D in our body is more than the recommended amount, there is a good chance that Vitamin D toxicity will follow.

Now, it is impossible for the amount of Vitamin D to go out of control in the body when the only real source is sun light. In our skin cells, the production of vitamin D is highly regulated. At the same speed as Vitamin D production, Vitamin D distribution also takes place. In addition to that, the amount of vitamin D produced in the skin with exposure to the sun is just about right for our body. So, being out in the sun should not be a matter of too much concern.

The only possibility of an overdose of Vitamin D is when we consume artificial sources of vitamin D. In most cases, it is the wrong dosage of Vitamin D supplement that leads to an overdose. There are some sure shot signs of vitamin D overdose including nausea and constipation. In cases of extreme overdose of Vitamin D it is possible that the rhythm of the heart gets altered. Kidney stone are another adverse consequence of Vitamin D overdose. Whenever you begin to consume supplements for Vitamin D, remember to watch out for these obvious signs. Studies have showed that almost all cases of Vitamin D toxicity are related to supplements. In other cases, there is a chance of over-consumption of cod liver oil that leads to this condition.

According to the recommendations of the Institute of Medicine, the safe amount of Vitamin D consumption per day is between 1500-2000 IU per day. In children and infants the level should never go beyond 1000 IU per day. This recommendation was made in the year 1997. However recent studies have led people to believe that the amount of Vitamin D supplementation required for the body is far beyond this recommended number. In the year 2010, the IOM brought out another study which revealed a drastic increase in the recommended levels.

According to this study, adults require 4000 IU of vitamin D each day while children can consume between 1000- 4000 IU per day depending upon their age. Another study revealed that adults can tolerate up to 10,000 IU each day. The debate is still on about this drastic increase in the recommended number.

However, the best way to balance your nutritional requirements is to avoid the theory of "more is better" in case of foods. Eat just what your body requires. In case your estimation is above or below this level, your body will show you signs early enough for you to restore normalcy.

Chapter 14: Treatment of Vitamin D Deficiency

Like any other nutritional deficit, it is mandatory that you check and treat any deficiency of vitamin D that may be present in your body. This is one of the easiest conditions to rectify if detected at an earlier stage. There are recommended treatment procedures that can be of great use to people who are suffering from Vitamin D deficiency induced problems.

The first and the most obvious step is to control the dietary intake of vitamin D. For those who have a deficiency, the recommended amount of vitamin D to correct the deficiency is predetermined. Of course, this number will vary depending upon the severity of the condition. Usually, when the blood level of Vitamin D is below 30 ng/ml, experts recommend a minimum intake of about 1000 IU/day in case of children. In adults who are suffering from vitamin D deficiency, the recommended daily intake is between 1500-2000IU per day.

There is a simple rule of thumb that will help you keep the amount of Vitamin D in the blood under control. For every 1ng/ml drop in the vitamin D level in the blood, you need to consume an additional 100 IU of vitamin per day.

According to a task force of the endocrine Society, the recommended daily intake for people who are suffering from Vitamin D deficiency is as follows:

- **Children in the age of 1-8 years**- These children can consume anything between 2000 IU of Vitamin D per day. The source of vitamin supplementation can come from Vitamin D3 or Vitamin D2 as per the preference of the child. This vitamin intake must be continued for at least 12 6 weeks with each week getting close to 50,000 IU of vitamin D. There is a maintenance therapy that is required after this period. During this period about 600 IU of Vitamin D must be provided to the child each day

- **For adults-** In case of adults who are suffering from a Vitamin D deficiency, it is necessary to consume at least 50,000IU of Vitamin D each week for about 8 weeks at a stretch. This intake is recommended to bring the Vitamin D level in the blood back to 30 ng/ml. The after therapy that is required to maintain the Vitamin D3 level requires at least 1000 IU of vitamin D per day.

- **Obese Individuals**- In obese individuals who may have the problem of malabsorption, it is extremely important to maintain the Vitamin D level at the recommended normal level. These individuals must consume at least 6000- 1000 IU each day to achieve the required 30 ng/.ml of Vitamin D.

Malabsorption is one of the most common problems faced by people who have a chronic case of Vitamin D deficiency in addition to consuming the recommended dietary levels of Vitamin D each day spending a few moments in the sun can do them a great deal of good in addition to that consuming vitamin rich foods like fatty fish, cod liver oil tablets and beef liver is highly recommended. It is possible to take preventive measures against Vitamin D deficiency a balanced diet and a healthy life style is the best way to keep yourself free from Vitamin D deficiency induced conditions.

It is very important for parents to ensure that children who are being exclusively breastfed should receive ample Vitamin D supplementation through either exposure to sunshine or through age appropriate fortified foods. It is during the formative years that Vitamin D deficiency is most likely to manifest itself. With necessary precautions and the right nutrition we can ensure healthy generations to come.

Conclusion

In my trials with nutrition, I have realized that our body is the best judge of what it requires. Everything that has developed in our body, including nutritional requirement is the result of several centuries of evolution. Hence, I believe that there is no better judge of what is right or wrong than the body itself. Now the only limitation in this whole equation is that we have learned to eat different things that are quite deviated from what is 'normal' and 'natural' for our body. Hence, we need to watch what we eat and eat right.

Take Vitamin D for example. This is a nutrient that has developed over time to manifest itself in several natural forms. In the beginning the only production of Vitamin D occurred in the ocean. When photosynthesis occurred in phytoplankton, vitamin D was produced. This was a process that started over 500 million years ago and continues to this date. The primitive forms of vertebrates were able to absorb the necessary amount of calcium from the ocean. They were able to get the required amount of Vitamin D by simply consuming plankton. When the vertebrates made their way on to land, they depended on an entirely different process. They had to consume Vitamin D from calcified remains of animals. It was only 350 million years ago that vertebrates made their own Vitamin D.

Considering that 350 million years ago is a long time, our bodies must have mastered the art of producing the required amount of Vitamin D in the body. So, in an ideal world, deficiency, supplementation and toxicity did not exist. But the truth is that we do not live in the ideal conditions.

Remember that we have our food on the go, spend most of our waking hours in cars or in our offices and obtain sunlight only from glass covered windows. How often do we take time in a day to step out in the sun? How often do we make it a conscious effort to consume the most natural and the healthiest foods available to us? How often do we think about the nutrition that the body is receiving?

If your answer is, not too often, my only hope is that this book has changed your mind. This book is not an attempt to just state the facts about Vitamin D. This is a manual that I have put together to help every single person think about what he or she is missing out on. The attempt is to help you understand that you might be putting yourself at the risk of unwanted disorders and health problems by not spending enough time on yourself.

Thank you again for downloading this book!

I hope this book was able to help you to learn how Vitamin D can benefit you in a number of different ways.

Here is a free preview of Digestive Health and Wellness: Clean Your Gut to Cure Disease, Strengthen Your Immune System and Heal Your Body

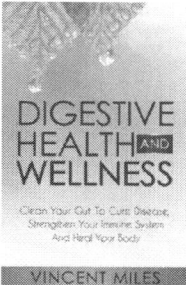

FREE PREVIEW Digestive Health and Wellness:

Chapter 1 A Holistic View on the Body

It is essential to clarify that a healthy gut is not only about assuring a fast digestion and having a good metabolism. True, keeping your gut clean will definitely result in the improvement of this part of your organism, but this is only one drop in the sea of overall effects that such a program will have.

A clean gut will improve both your physical and your mental state, since you will feel fresher and stronger. Weight loss is another significant result of maintaining an effective digestion through eating healthy. Your overall energy levels will change and psychologically you'll find you have a more vibrant state of mind, you feel much lighter in your body movements, you enjoy better concentration capacity, and a visible energy boost that will give you the strength you need in your daily activities.

Dr. Eva Cwynar, author of *The Fatigue Solution*, has already emphasized the role played by the digestive track in improving your general energy levels and performance. She recommends eating a lot of proteins in the morning, having small meals every 3-4 hours, and picking up mostly fresh fruit and vegetables, nuts and cereals as well as cheese and meat for your diet. In her opinion, all this will lead to a much better mood and overall capacity of your organism, as you'll be eating for energy, not for calories.

Dr. Alejandro Junger in his famous book *Clean Gut* goes even further and explains his belief that a dirty gut is at the root of all our health problems, even though we may not know it or we may only notice one link in the whole chain (a surface one), only one aspect in the overall dynamics of reactions that take place in our body. He considers the gut to be at the root of all disease if our digestion is left unchecked. It is wide known that severe diseases such as cancer, diabetes, autoimmune diseases, and even heart disease can be traced back to gut disorders. However what many of us may not be aware of is that even lighter forms of illness such as mood swings, constipation, fatigue, eczema, or low libido are caused by a less than perfect functioning of our digestive system ... at least to a certain extent. Of course there are myriad other disease causes, just as numerous as the sources of toxins we're exposed to nowadays! Aging is also a natural course and it is true that our body defenses weaken as time goes by. Naturally you would hardly think your libido is affected by the food you eat when you're over 50 and you don't feel as young and bouncy as you once did. Maybe you don't, but you can try to feel livelier and a healthy diet is one of the recommendable ways to go. A healthy gut is one of your main weapons in trying to slow down or attenuate the effects of aging. You will certainly not find any ambrosia or elixir for eternal life, but you can help your body stay young, more energetic and healthier for a longer while.

Did you know that, more or less literally, about two thirds of your immune system is in your gut? Your gut is like an ecosystem, with its varied flora of bacteria that help you process food you ingest, regulate digestion and hormones, excrete toxins, and produce vitamins or other compounds. Nature works according to an inner logic that is obviously extremely operative and simultaneously so discrete, that we can barely grasp it under normal circumstances. When something goes out of balance, we become aware of dysfunction. However more often than not it is hard to acknowledge that it may very well is something unwillingly provoked by us through our eating habits and carelessness towards our organism. If the natural order in that ecosystem runs out of balance, the whole organism is likely to suffer and this in turn will have disruptive effects on your performance as an individual in many respects.

Picture a diaphanous convoluted chord in your body. That is the brain-gut connection. It's not immediately evident, because we learned to separate and evaluate the functions in our organism according to different systems whose activity appears quite independent. In reality our body works in concordance with an ingenious mechanism whose main force resembles electric current. When there's an energetic deficit due to disease or disorder in your gut, the flow to and in your brain will also be affected. Anatomically speaking, this connection between the gut and the brain explains why you can feel nausea or indigestion after you take antidepressants, why you can get depressive or get headache if you have bad digestion, why you either overeat, or you can't eat at all when you feel anxious, stressed out, sad, or terribly preoccupied with some problem. Even the butterflies in your stomach when you are in love or infatuated reflect this deep organic connection that we usually ignore. When you have to speak in public or to go on stage, why do you think you feel something shivering at the level of your gut, too? Because of this intrinsic connection between these two areas of your organism; sensitivity in one place reverberates in the other.

The bottom line is that some disease causes are easier to control and this is definitely the case when it comes to the health of our gut. Moreover, just as we should adopt a holistic take on your health; it's much better if we think long-term. When it comes to food, it's is without any doubt not easy to think of staying healthy ten years from now when you have a steaming steak in front of you or when your friend invites you to a cruelly tempting Pizza alla Diavola. Yes, you may feel you have to grab that hamburger in your break from work and get back to something serious fast. But as mature beings, if we can create some order in our lives, why not do it? It takes a great deal of determination and force of will, that's for sure. We also have to be very aware of the actual consequences of our impulsive eating: when we yield to a savory temptation, it's not only about feeling a bit bloated for the rest of the day or 'gaining' a pound or two. It's actually about making a decision about how much health you allow yourself to have in the future and even long you want the rest of your life to be. In other words, our diet is also about treasuring our bodies and about practicing love for ourselves.

Printed in Great Britain
by Amazon